The
Basic Keys
To
Healthy Living

A Practical Guide To General Wellness

Abraham Mkpe

TABLE OF CONTENTS

Introduction

There are different categories of health challenges that people of different calibers and status grapple with throughout their life time, some of these health issues result to incapacitation and death.

However, majority of such health issues could have been absolutely averted if the relevance of safety consciousness healthy living was properly and timely conceptualized.

It is highly pertinent for you to always remain conscious of the fact that your healthy living is highly essential to your efficient, productive and effective existence, and therefore, be absolutely committed to doing what it takes to achieve a healthy life.

That is, if you must enjoy the purpose of your existence, coupled with being a blessing to your world, rather than being a burden and a liability, the concept of taking safety consciousness as a necessary measure required for safeguarding your healthy living must not be taken for granted.

Health challenges are major channels by which many people spend a large proportion of their earnings and resources in this our contemporary world.

This menace of wasting a very large proportion of one's resources on health related issues could be drastically minimized if only people become more sensitized, and also have proper concept about the need to take safety consciousness with all seriousness.

In our world today, we are unavoidably poised with the challenges of being exposed to various degrees of health hazards, emanating from environmental pollution, water pollution, air pollution, noisy environments, congestion, scientific exploration and experimentation, climate change and so on.

These and many other factors had made many people to be consistently confronted with different categories of health hazards, many of which could result to life time challenges and many result to incapacitation or even death.

Being that as it may, in order to ensure that the degree to which we grapple with avoidable health issues is minimized, it is then required on our own part to ensure the proper and timely application of certain key information, so as to be able to avert gripping health challenges that can make life unbearable and a threat to human existence.

In this highly resourceful book, we shall be navigating some basic keys that are highly essential to reducing the risks of health hazards, consistent and timely application of these safety nuggets will eventually translate into attaining and living a healthy life.

These basic keys include living a life of total obedience to God. It's quite evident that disobedience to God is highly disastrous and calamitous, deliberately disobeying God can put someone in the state of perpetual ill health.

To avert the calamity of perpetual sickness and all conditions of ill health, you must ensure that iniquity, which is an aspect of disobedience to God, as matter of a necessity is completely avoided.

Another important key to healthy living as we are going to be discussing in this book is the key of safety consciousness.

This is a highly essential key to healthy living that many people have taken for granted. Lack of safety consciousness makes your life to be highly susceptible to diverse degrees of health hazards.

In this book, we shall also be looking at the importance of personal hygiene as it concerns our healthy living. Ideally, taking personal hygiene for granted while expecting a miracle to happen in your health life is child's play.

We shall furthermore look at another essential key that is highly significant to healthy living in this book, and that is the importance of knowing your genetic nature.

You must never forget that understanding of your genetic nature is highly essential to your healthy living.

Furthermore, we shall also be taking a critical look at the significance of developing and maintaining a positive habit in relation to achieving a healthy life.

It's absolutely an undeniable fact that, many health challenges that people grapple with without any possible solution are directly traceable to negative life styles.

Another essential key to a healthy living as we shall see in this book is that of our habitat, our environment. It is evident that people's health lives are measured to some extent by the nature of their environment. That is to say your health to some extent is a product of your environment.

More so, we shall be taking a critical look at the essential of routine medical checkups in relation to our health. One the major importance of routine medical checkups is early detection of health issues in the body system and prompt action.

Lastly, in the context of this book, we shall be taking a critical examination of the relevance of exercise to our healthy living. We shall also examine the different kinds of exercises that would be suitable for individuals depending on their body chemistry and health history.

If your health life is valuable and essential to you, if you really desire to live a healthy life that eventually translates to longevity, then you will need to settle down with this book, digest all the information, develop a life of health safety consciousness, and you will definitely see a robust boost in your health life.

Chapter One

TOTAL OBEDIENCE TO GOD

Biblically, illness is associated with the expression of God's total displeasure toward an individual, family or nation as a result of an act of outright disobedience God, which could be by way of iniquity, trespass, transgression or sin.

God could use the expression of the disposition of His displeasure toward peoples' immoral attitudes both as punitive and corrective measures, just to ensure that man is brought back to the path of sanity and righteousness.

It is quite obvious that God does not derive any form of pleasure or fulfillment in watching people go through any form of illness or discomfort. That is absolutely not God's nature; He derives zero pleasure in people's plight.

However, due to man's continuous act of willful disobedience to God right from the time of creation, God sometimes deliberately allow men to be afflicted with diverse degrees of health challenges including death in some instances.

Man in The Garden Of Eden

God created man in His image and likeness, unlike every other creatures, man had the express nature of God to reasonable degree.

While man was still in the Garden of Eden, he was freely enjoying virtually everything because; sin has not entered into the world.

There was nothing like famine, no laborious work, no trading, no business, no stress of any kind, no pain, and there was no illness of any kind at all.

The only assignment given to them by God then was "to dress the Garden and to keep it." Genesis 2:15.

Afterward, God gave man a very simple instruction on what to eat in the Garden and what he should not eat.

However, it is a pity that of all the trees that God gave man access to as food, including the tree of life; man completely ignored everything and rather chose to walk in outright disobedience to the instruction given to him by God. Genesis 2:15, 16, 17.

From the moment man disobeyed God, by eating of the fruit of the tree of the knowledge of good and evil, contrary to God's word, man has not been able to get it right with God.

That singular act of disobedience has put man in the perpetual condition of grappling with all manner of discomforts from generation to generation.

The Fall Of Man

Man's disobedience to God in the Garden of Eden by eating the fruit of the tree of knowledge of good and evil has completely changed the narrative of God's plan and purpose for mankind. Genesis 3:6-7, 9-13

The Consequences Of The Fall of Man

i.   *Sorrow In Conception*

It is absolutely undisputable that majority of the ill health conditions that women go through during conception, including the stress, the pain of labor, delivery and maternal mortality in some cases are as a result of the consequences of disobeying God.

ii.   *The Pain Of Childbirth*

The devil continually capitalizes on the curse that was pronounced on Eve as a result of her disobedience to God; and also for influencing Adam to also disobey God, to keep enforcing the curse of having sorrow in childbirth on women during their labor and delivery.

That was never part of God's plan for man when he was created, without the sin of disobedience, women would have been given birth without any trace of pain.

iii.   *Cursed Is The Ground*

Although God did not make a direct pronouncement of curse on Adam, however, the ground was cursed for the sake of man. That is, the reason why God was cursing the earth was to enable it have negative bearings on the life of man.

God declared to man, in sorrow shall you eat of it all the days of your life. That means, man will live a perpetual life of sorrow, illness, pain, discomforts, etc.

The ground will no more be productive in commensurate to the labor and efforts of man. In addition to that, unlike before, man now has to labor before he can eat, compared with when he was still in the Garden of Eden, where everything was readily available.

"Thou shall eat herbs of the field". As a result of the curse that emanated from man's disobedience to God, the originally prepared diet for man was also swapped from fruits to herbs, compared with when he was still living in obedience to God.

Man now had to labor and struggle for survival all the days of his life, that wasn't the plan of God when he created man, all these discomforts came as a result of man's willful disobedience to God.

Disobedience to God resulted to making man to end up experiencing all sort of labor, distress, struggle, all forms of pains and will have to face all form of challenges and will eventually have to die, all these are the direct consequences of disobedience to God.

Furthermore, disobedience to God also resulted to preventing man from having access to the tree of life, which was originally his right.

Man was consequently sent out of the blissful Garden in order to totally prevent him from having any access to the tree of life.

Disobedience to God resulted to man's expulsion from his beautiful home, the Garden of Eden, his peaceful habitation, where he never had to labor to enjoy the essential things of life, where every need had been made available ever before he was created.

Disobedience, The Genesis of Unhealthy Living

The abnormality of Cain killing Abel his brother was one of the major consequences of Adam's disobedience to God in the Garden of Eden.

If Cain was really normal and not mentally deranged, he wouldn't have ever considered killing his own brother after God had rejected him and his offering.

Ordinarily, what a sane person would have done was to prepare another offering that would be acceptable to God, and not seeing killing Abel as a means to console himself for his rejection.

Killing Abel will in no wise make God to reconsider Cain or his offering, that action rather took him to another dimension of God's displeasure.

Knowing that Cain had murdered Abel because God accepted him and his offering was must have impacted the lives of Adam and Eve in a negative way. The news must have affected them both emotionally and psychologically.

Also coupled with the fact of hearing the judgment that God has pronounced on Cain that he was going to be a fugitive and vagabond, all due to their disobedience to God. All these must have taken a negative toll on their general wellness.

Cain was not spared at all for killing his brother, his action was a grievous act of iniquity against God and humanity, therefore, he was made to face the consequence squarely, in addition to the curse that was already pronounce on the ground for the sake of man.

There was no way Cain would have evaded the consequences of his evil act because, the blood of his brother, whom he had gruesomely murdered was crying against him for vengeance to the extent that God couldn't ignore.

Cain was cursed directly: One of curse that was declared on Cain was that the earth, which has opened its mouth to receive the blood of Abel shall no more yield commensurate result to Cain's labor and efforts.

Cain was also cursed with a health condition similar to that of insanity; he became a fugitive and a vagabond.

The LORD Plagued Pharaoh

Apart from the words fugitive and vagabond, which are believed to have some traits or elements of mental incapacitation, the first place the word associated directly to illness is mentioned in the Scripture is in Genesis 12:17, where the Bible records that God plagued (afflict, scourge) king Pharaoh of Egypt together with his entire house hold with great plagues (great afflictions).

Pharaoh the king of Egypt took Sarah, Abraham's wife, although not really knowing that the woman was married to Abraham, yet it was considered as a breach against God's standard, since the woman was someone's wife.

It is therefore quite evident that, every act of disobedience to God in form of transgression, iniquity, trespass, injustice, corruption or any form of sin, has the capability of attracting God's anger or displeasure and consequently ill health conditions.

The fact that the consequence did not manifest immediately does not change the reality of the fact that, outright disobedience to God in any way will always have their attendant negative consequences.

Plagues Against Pharaoh And Egypt

When king Pharaoh together with his people refused to allow the children of Israel to go out of the land of Egypt in accordance with God's instruction, God decided to plague the house of king Pharaoh together with the entire land of Egypt.

It is quite obvious from the biblical point of view that, whenever anyone or a group of people decide to despise God's instruction and walk in disobedience to Him, there is always a repercussion.

It does not really matter whether you are a child of God or not, it is obvious that God expects everyone to walk in total obedience to Him, anything contrary to this will always bring grievous consequences, whether sooner or later.

Some of the major reasons why God always ensure that people face the consequences of their disobedience to Him include the following:

a. So as to enable people to walk in the fear God.
b. It is a means of curbing disobedience against God.
c. To prevent impunity and serve as deterrence.
d. It proves that God is a God of justice and not a respecter of men.

Disobedience Brings Curses And Unhealthy Living

While obedience to God produces blessings from God, ranging from the blessing of joy, rest, progress, favor, promotion, victory, sound health, fruitfulness, increase, enlargement, greatness, prosperity, abundance etc.

It is evident that all these kind of physical and spiritual blessings of God on a man's life have the capacity of making it possible for one to achieve a robust healthy living.

On the contrary, living in willful disobedience to God attracts His displeasure and curses upon man, which on the long run makes life totally unbearable.

The curses that emanate from outright disobedience to God include perpetual sorrow, failure, shame, defeat, stagnation, limitation, frustration, adversity, lack, retrogression, demotion, bondage, reproach, poverty, depression, rejection, and so on and so forth.

The resultant effect of these curses in a man's life is inability to live and achieve a robust healthy life.

It will surprise you that the majority of diverse health conditions that different people grapple with in life today without any possible solution are mentioned in connection with the curses of disobeying God. Deuteronomy 28:19-22, 27-28, 60-61.

The Jews' Concept of Consequences of Disobedience

The Israelites were very much familiar with the reality of the fact that one of the common factors responsible for man's plight in form of any kind of ill health condition is willful disobedience to God, summed up as sin.

This was simply because sin was the common cause of sickness in the Bible days. It was quite clear in their days that sin against God always attracted the display of His utter displeasure in form of all manner of ill health conditions.

In the days of Jesus Christ, after healing a man that was having an infirmity for the period of thirty eight years. Right there, Jesus knew that sin was directly responsible for his thirty eight year old ill health condition.

After a while, Jesus Christ met him in the Temple on another occasion and admonished him and said to him "See, you are well again. Stop sinning or something worse may happen to you". John 5:14

This is a very clear indication to the fact that there is a correlation between sin, which is summed up as total disobedience to God and illness.

It was also on the back drop of this understanding of the Jews that the disciples of Jesus Christ enquired from Him in order to ascertain whose sin was responsible for the ill health condition of a particular man that was born blind, the man or his parents. John 9:1-3.

Jesus Christ however clarified this by telling them that, although iniquity is an invitation to calamity, nevertheless, the man's plight of being born blind was not as a result of sin factor, that neither he nor his parents were responsible.

That is, even though, disobedience to God is capable of attracting all manner of ill health conditions, however, it is evident that it's not all health challenges that emanate from disobedience to God.

Chapter Two

SAFETY CONSCIOUSNESS

God created man in such a wonderful and excellent manner that he's created with certain potentials of being able to determine the things that should happen around him and the ones that should not happen.

It will then amount to nothing but foolishness of the highest order on man's part, when one begins to expect God or His angels to do for him those things he had being empowered to do by himself.

There are certain basic things such as taking the full responsibilities of safety consciousness, which should be your sole duty and not that of God or of His angels. God expects us to trust Him for the things we can't do by ourselves and not for the ones He had fully empowered us to do for ourselves and by ourselves.

You can trust and depend on God for instance in situations whereby you have absolutely limited abilities, or when you have completely done that which is your own responsibilities.

Your failure to fully deploy your efforts with the wisdom God has given you and keep claiming you're walking in faith is nothing but tempting God. That is not an act of faith, it is neither an act trusting God, that is rather an act of foolishness and tempting God.

Under this topic, we shall be looking at safety consciousness as regards the necessary and required safety steps to be taken in order to safeguard the hazards to our physical health.

Evidently, safety consciousness is highly essential to a healthy living, your negligence to these key factor, as far as your health is concerned is nothing but unnecessarily exposing yourself to the risks of frequent health challenges, incapacitation and premature death.

Some highly essential key safety consciousness which can translate into a healthy living and longevity among other benefits include the following:

1. *Avoiding Unnecessary Risks*

For instance, taking the risk of fumigating with highly concentrated chemicals such as insecticides, herbicides, germicides etc, which are highly inimical to your health, with the erroneous concept of it doesn't matter, or God will protect me, is not faith but foolishness, tempting God and exposing yourself to avoidable dangerous and deadly health hazards.

That's not how faith works, that is negligence, foolishness and tempting God. Inhaling just a little quantity of such substance from time to time could lead to a very severe life time health challenge, incapacitation or even sudden death.

As a sprayer, whether spraying of vehicles, woodwork, etc, it's highly essential for you to be conscious of the fact that you're dealing with dangerous chemicals that could be highly inimical to your general wellness.

Therefore, you must as a matter of necessity consistently imbibe the culture of safety consciousness by ensuring that you're always protecting yourself from inhaling any quantity of those chemicals.

Inhaling just a little quantity of those chemicals could lead to damaging some critical and sensitive body organs like the lungs, heart, liver, kidney etc. Apart from the risks related to inhaling the chemicals, direct contact with your eye or your skin could also be hazardous.

A little and constant consciousness of the hazards that this chemicals pose to your health will go a very long way in enabling you to always take proactive measures against anything that is a hazard to your healthy living.

Essentially, you should cultivate the habit of the consciousness of ensuring that no quantity of any of these dangerous chemicals, whether cement, paints, insecticides, germicides, herbicides or whatever chemicals find their way into your sensitive organs or systems.

This is a very highly essential way to maintain a healthy living, protecting your health is far cheaper and easier than trying to procure health after it had been tampered with.

Above all, if your job is the type that unavoidably exposes you to certain health hazards without any provision to safeguard your health, wisdom demands that you should quit such a job for the purpose of safeguarding your life.

What is the essence of a job that has become a threat to your health and your life, what is the essence of a job when you eventually spend all your earnings on medication at the end of the day?

Remember, if you don't quit while you are still very strong and healthy, by the time the risks and the hazards of the job eventually overwhelm your effectiveness and your productivity, you will lose your job on the long run and may eventually lose your life. Therefore make the hale while sun shines.

2. The Relevance of Safety Kits

Except where and when it has become extremely unavoidable, there should be no reason or excuses for not wearing a life jacket if you must travel by water. The right thing has to be done, safety first.

Even if you can swim very well, then wearing your life jacket will serve as an added advantage to you in case of any eventuality.

It is an undeniable fact that safety is of the Lord. However, it will be reasonable for you to use your initiatives by wearing your life jacket if you must use water transportation, and then allow God to do His own part.

For instance, one of the importance of making use of life jacket to you in case of boat accident is that, whether you know how to swim or not, with the aid of your life jacket on, you remain afloat without much stress, at least for a while until rescuers will come your way, depending on the type of the water way.

Then if you can swim, it makes it even easier; you keep floating with less stress.

However, when you don't put on your life jacket and you don't know how to swim at all, in case of any boat accident; it is not easy to rescue you in the first place, compared with someone with his life jacket on, because you are not floating.

Secondly, when you don't put on your life jacket and an accident occurs, in a very short time, you are sinking and unwillingly drinking water, and that makes it very easy for you to sink and die because of the intake of excessive water.

Many people have lost their lives prematurely when such deaths could have been totally averted, just because of their lack of safety consciousness that makes people to take unnecessary risk at the expense of their life, when they should have taken very simple and safe safety and precautionary measures.

3. *Essentials of Abstinence*

Abstinence in this context has to do with completely staying away from anything that is capable of triggering health challenges in your life. No matter how delightful or pleasurable such a thing may be, if it constitutes health hazard, you must help yourself by totally abstaining from it.

In other words, there is a dire need for you to properly understand your body chemistry's reaction to certain things such as weather, food, cream, soap, perfumes etc.

Whenever you discover that you're allergic to a particular thing, you don't need to develop affection for such a thing but rather avoid it for the sake of your health.

Therefore, settle down and find out the things that trigger health challenges in your life and make sure you avoid such things completely. Adopting the principle of prevention is better than cure will help you a lot in this regards.

For instance, cold weather and cold drinks have the capability of triggering pneumonia; stuffy environment or smoke can also trigger asthmatic condition.

Essentially, wisdom demands that completely abstaining from anything that is capable of triggering any health challenge in your life must be a regular practice.

4. *Importance of Nose Mask*

Before the outbreak of COVID 19 pandemic, and the subsequent mandatory introduction of the use of nose mask globally as recommended by the World Health Organization (WHO), nose mask usage was exclusively reserved to the health workers and some other food handlers.

The most popular and common nose mask was then known as the surgical mask.

However, as result of the outbreak of COVID 19 epidemic, nose mask was recommended as a key preventive measure against the spread of the virus. This was owing to the fact that it was discovered that COVID could majorly be contacted through saliva, via mouth to mouth or nose to mouth.

After sometime, it was discovered that using nose mask can also prevent people from contacting other infections that could be communicated through saliva or coughing.

For the fear of contacting COVID 19, everybody became a user of nose mask for the purpose of prevention. The laws of "no nose mask, no entry" was everywhere. No one was entitled to enjoying any service without wearing nose mask.

Today, just because the law of "no nose mask, no entry" is relaxed, people that should ordinarily use nose mask for their personal safety and hygiene have also relaxed.

When you know the importance of using nose mask as a necessary safety measure for safeguarding your health, you won't wait for anyone to enforce any law on you before you start to do what is necessary and essential.

There is no price too much to pay for safety purpose, and there's nothing too much to do in order to ensure you're taking the necessary safety measures that will eventually translate to making it possible for you to experience a viable healthy life.

5. Necessary Preventive Measures

If you're doing a job that exposes you to certain health challenges like welding for instance, it could be your personal job or what you are employed to do, make sure you're health safety conscious, and ensure to take safety measures by always wearing your welding glasses to protect your eyes.

Don't wait for God or expect God to take your responsibility for you, when He has given you all the wisdom that you need to take preventive measures.

Make sure you always take every simple and necessary preventive measure to ensure that you don't expose any part of your body to any form of harm or damage.

Protecting yourself from certain hazards is a way of avoiding unnecessary spending on health related challenges.

Your safety consciousness is a way of completely safeguarding yourself from health related challenges that have plunged many people into frequently spending their resources on drugs, which could have been completely avoided.

The failure to take safety consciousness with all seriousness on the part of some people has resulted to incurring incurable diseases. Moreover, this failure on the part of others had resulted to incapacitation or untimely death.

6. *Personal Protective Equipment*

There are some jobs that require the mandatory use of all personal protective equipment in order to ensure that your basic safety is guaranteed.

In such a situation, the need for the use of such required protective kits should not be seen by you as a burden or as optional when you take safety consciousness with all seriousness.

As a matter of fact, when you are working in a place where your safety is not a concern to your employer, it is wise that you quit such a job. No one should take your health safety for granted, and no one should be more conscious about the safety of your health than yourself.

Making use of your safety kits may not always be convenient, however when you consider the importance of the safety of your health to your life, you will always choose to make use of your kits to ensure your overall safety.

Make use of all your personal protective kits where it is required; use your safety boot, safety helmet, your nose mask, your coverall, your hand gloves etc. All these kits are recommended as safety measures to safeguard you from certain health hazards.

If you're working in a place where you're unavoidably exposed to certain health hazards, make sure your personal protective kids that have been given to you are not ignored for whatever reason, except whereby using them constitutes another threat to your health.

7. *The Relevance of Seat Belts*

The use of seat belts in cars, buses or airplanes may not be one hundred percent safe, but considerably, I think making use of your seat belt in this regards has more advantage than disadvantages.

Some people are so ignorant about the importance of using the seat belt as a safety measure to cushion the effect of accident to the extent that, the only reason they use it is to avoid been seeing as breaking the traffic rules.

Many people's reason for not making use of seat belt is because they are of the opinion that using seat belt is not totally safe and has its own disadvantages. This may be correct to certain extent, but the disadvantages can't be compared with the advantages.

If we consider it from the optimistic point of view, we can simply conclude that no matter what, the advantages of making use of seat belt as a safety measure in cushioning the effects of accident far out weights the disadvantages that one can ever imagine.

8. Helmet/Safety Caps

There are some places where you can't ride your motor bikes without making use of helmet or safety cap, this not just for the purpose of making laws, it is a way of ensuring that proactive measures that guarantee certain level of safety are taken in case of any crash.

Ironically, in many other societies, nobody cares whether you make use of your safety cap or helmet or not, you are on your own.

Pathetically, such people riding motor bikes without taking any safety measure by making use of helmet or safety caps and unavoidably exposing themselves to health hazards would be subjected to paying taxes to the authority for owning and making use of motor bikes.

Ideally, whether or not there is a law mandating you to make use of helmet or safety cap, wisdom demands that you should use your own discretion to ensure that you take every necessary safety measure against anything that is capable of jeopardizing your health.

Your greatest and most valuable asset and wealth that must be discretely and properly guarded is your health. Remember, your health is your wealth, therefore do everything that is required to protect it.

Protecting your health by consistently taking simple and necessary safety measures is far cheaper than trying to restore it after it has been tampered with due to your negligence to safety consciousness.

9. Genotype

Having a sense of safety consciousness will enable you to understand the importance of knowing your genotype. There are many people who don't bother about the need for them to know their genotype and also their blood group.

One of the major reasons why it is a necessity to have adequate knowledge of genotype among many other reasons is for the purpose of preventing your children from experiencing the debilitating scourge of sickle cell anemia.

For instance, if as a man you don't know that your genotype is A/S and you went ahead to marry someone who also does not know that her genotype is A/S, if both of you have two or three children together, the tendency of one or more of your children having sickle cell anemia is very high.

This is a very simple health challenge that could be totally prevented when there is proper awareness for safety consciousness. But because of lack of proper safety consciousness awareness, many people have been trapped by this scourge of totally preventable health condition.

As a result of people's a poor attitude towards safety consciousness, this simple act of negligence has eventually resulted to situations of life time regrets, marital crisis, continuous battle with the health of the affected children and loss of children in many cases.

Chapter Three

PERSONAL HYGIENE

Maintaining your physical and mental health depends majorly on a qualitative practice of personal hygiene, which is the bedrock of your daily life. The act of always keeping yourself clean and taking proper care of your body is the premise upon which good and proper healthy living is predicated.

Personal hygiene are a collection of certain practices you may adopt on the daily basis for the purpose of improving your health, and this eventually translate into achieving a robust healthy living and longevity.

The majority of these practices revolve round always keeping your environment tidy and making yourself neat and presentable.

The simple practice of regular bathing, hand washing, dental care, hair care, and nails care are all part of maintaining good personal hygiene.

These are daily practices that may not really look inspiring but are of immense significance for keeping one healthy, averting damaging of your body parts and ensuring longevity.

Personal hygiene is not just about looking good, that is to say, personal hygiene goes beyond the overall notion of regarding it as just an ordinary way to make you look good.

Rather, personal hygiene also implies tidying up your environment, taking good care of yourself, respecting yourself; preventing yourself from becoming endangered to avoidable illnesses and ensuring you remain healthy.

1. Hand Washing

The simple habit of regular hand washing is one of the highly essential routines in the pursuance of personal hygiene. However, this practice may appear to be very effortless; nevertheless, it is a highly essential instrument in combating the spread of dangerous and deadly diseases.

This very simple act of washing your hands frequently will go a long way in helping you to achieve getting rid of bacteria and virus that you may have unwittingly come in contact with in the course of your daily activities, and in the course of your interaction with people.

The act of regular hand washing is highly essential to maintaining personal hygiene, especially before meals and after using the bathroom.

Effective Procedures For Hand Washing.

i.   It is highly ideal and more effective to use warm water and soap for not less than twenty seconds.

ii. It is also important to make a hand sanitizer available for situations where soap and water cannot be easily gotten.

iii. One of the most effective ways to wash your hands is to ensure it is done under running water.

iv. While washing your hands, ensure you scrub between your fingers and under your nails properly.

Hand washing has social relevance in addition to the obvious health benefits in the sense that in most cases, people with clean and tidy hands are more likely to be trusted and approached.

When To Wash Your Hands

i.   Always make sure you wash your hands immediately after using the toilet to enable you get rid of any possible fecal contamination.

ii.   Hand washing is highly essential before and after eating or handling food.

iii. Ensure to wash your hands properly after changing diapers, this is very important.

iv.   It's also very important to wash your hands before and after caring for a sick person or cleaning up bodily fluids.

v.   Hand washing is necessary before and after tending to cuts or wounds, that is, before and after administering first aids to a patient or injured person.

vi.   Always wash your hands after blowing your nose; this is highly essential to your health and that of others around you.

vii.   After touching trash, dirty surfaces, objects, or corpses; after doing some cleaning, it is essential to wash your hands.

viii.   Wash your hands after handling pets or farm animals to prevent the spread of germs.

ix.   It is highly essential and hygienic to always wash your hands after visiting clinics or hospitals.

x.   It is also necessary to wash your hands after handling chemicals.

2. Dental Care

Maintaining good dental hygiene is highly essential to your dental health and your overall health. Brushing and flossing twice a day will go a long way in preventing dental related problems such as mouth odor, gum disease, tooth loss, cavities, in addition to freshening your breath.

It has been proven that negligence to your dental health and hygiene increases your risk of developing acute diseases like diabetes, and heart diseases.

Moreover, whenever you have tooth ache, your head also aches.

Dental Care Tips

i. Always brush your teeth at least twice a day, especially after dinner or before going to bed.
ii. Don't forget to clean your tongue and use mouth wash.
iii. Gaggling your mouth with warm water mixed with little salt is highly essential for dental care and health.
iv. Regular dental checkup is very essential for preventive care and early detection of dental problems.

The relevance of your dental hygiene and care must not be neglected when it comes to the issue of keeping yourself clean and healthy.

3. Hair Care

Another critical area of personal hygiene that must not be taken for granted as far as your health is concerned is taking proper care of your hair. It is evident that taking proper and regular care for your hair is of immense significant to your health, and to your looking good as well.

Obviously, apart from its relevance to enhancing your physical appearance, your clean, neat, and properly treated hair also have a way of improving your comfort and health.

For instance, when you consistently maintain a clean, dandruff free scalp with constant shampooing and conditioning, it translates to enabling to keep you looking your best, as well as maintaining a regular trimming and styling.

Tips For Hair Care

i. It is very important for you to always ensure you are using the proper type of shampooing and conditions that are appropriate for your hair type.

ii. You must always try as much as possible to shun immoderate use of heating appliances to keep you from inflicting any possible hurt to your scalp.

iii. It is highly essential and hygienic to get a regular trimming in order to maintain healthy hair.

As a result of the profound influence that hair hygiene might impact on both your psychological and emotional condition, it is imperative that you should never underrate this highly essential aspect of your habit for practicing self-care.

As a matter of fact, the need for taking proper care of your hair as a way of maintaining personal hygiene cannot be over emphasized.

4. Skin Care

It is obvious that skin care hygiene is a highly essential aspect of personal hygiene that is goes far beyond the measure of simple concerns about appearance.

There is a dire need to always maintain a healthy skin that would be characterized with utmost flexibility and free from any trait of skin disorders.

The simple and regular practice of washing, hydrating, moisturizing and protecting your skin from the damaging effects of the sun and environmental pollutants are the major components of an effective skincare habit.

Steps For Skincare

i. Fundamentally, it is highly essential for you to properly understand your skin type. That is, there is a need for you to have a proper understanding of your skin nature, and then ensure to apply only the appropriate and applicable products that are suitable for your skin.

ii. Always ensure to make do with sunscreen in order to safeguard your skin from ultra violet damage.

iii. Ensure you conscientiously develop the practice of a consistent skin care routine because of the great significance of your skin to your general wellness.

In addition to the overall advantages of your physical health that skin care provides, it also enhances your overall psychological and emotional wellness.

When you feel absolutely good about how you look, it can have a favorable impact on many different facets of your life, from the quality of your personal relationships to your ability to advance professionally.

5. Nail Care

Evidently, your pursuance of personal hygiene will definitely not be fully achieved without the need for a proper nail care being fully included.

As a matter of fact, this highly essential aspect of hygiene has been underrated and neglected by many, forgetting the reality of the fact that disregarding the need for nail care while seeking to achieve personal hygiene is nothing but deflating one's efforts for achieving a robust healthy living.

A proper maintenance for your nails has a very important part to play in preventing the spread of infectious bacteria and germs, and at the same time guaranteeing achieving a healthy life.

Nail care is of immense significance to your health and hygiene, always keeping them clean and trimmed is also optimal for looking good.

Nail Care Tips

i.   Always keep your nails clean and prevent them from being constantly wet, this will enable you in a great way to safeguard you from contracting fungal infections.

ii.   In order to prevent the spread of germs make sure you avoid biting your nails.

iii.   To avoid hurtful nail breakages, enable to trim your nails and file them regularly.

Your continuous nonchalant attitudes to the significance of the care of your nails can culminate in problems like fungal infections and the buildup of dirt and bacteria, which are easily communicable to your mouth or other parts of your body.

Always be conscious of the reality of the fact that periodic maintenance of nails health is of great importance for both your wellbeing as an individual and also that of everyone around you.

The Benefits Of Personal Hygiene

The act of practicing good hygiene has enormous benefits; the effects are personal hygiene are far more than just your body, it has far reaching consequences. Some of the benefits of consistently maintaining and practicing personal hygiene include the followings:

I.   *Disease Prevention*

One of the major of advantage of practicing personal hygiene routine is that of enabling you to successfully attain the prevention of contacting infectious diseases.

The personal hygiene behavior of periodic hand washing, general washings of dirty clothes, dishes, sinks, bath, toilet, dental maintenance and overall cleanliness will go a very long way in enabling you to minimize the possibility of contracting dangerous viruses and germs.

II.   *Improved Self Esteem*

The act of keeping yourself clean and tidy can do a lot of surprises for your sense of propriety and honor. When you have a sense of feeling good about your appearance, it gives you a sense of enthusiasm and optimism on the rest of your life.

III.   *An Enhanced Social Intervention*

Sustaining a high value of a lifestyle of personal hygiene has extra rewards apart from merely carrying good appearance and feeling better. Interactions with others are improved when you maintain a clean and presentable appearance.

IV.   *An Enhanced Mental Wellness*

Sustaining a consistent hygienic exercise is one way to improve your psychological health. It enhances a reassuring confidence. Your positive approach toward life and your capability to deal with life challenges will both be improved when you look clean and refreshed.

V.   *Qualitative Sleep*

It is highly essential to improve the quality of your sleep by making sure you thoroughly make yourself clean before bed.

Making sure your body is clean and also imbibing the habit of putting on night wears will enable you to have a good sleep, which in turn will enable you to wake up with enthusiasm and optimism fully prepared to take on the day.

VI.   *Increased Productivity*

Being completely delighted in one's neatness and enjoying the reinvigorated strength that accompanies it translates into getting more done. It helps you zero in on the basic task at hand, whether it is work related or personal.

Maintaining adequate general body cleanliness enhances psychological focus and wellness which eventually translates into enhancing productive action.

VII. *Preventing Body Odor*

One of the greatest benefits you derive from maintaining a life of personal hygiene is achieving a body that is completely free from odor. In most cases, body odor is a product of lack of personal hygiene; personal hygiene is highly essential to healthy living.

When you keep putting in the required energy to ensure attaining good hygiene, you have succeeded in applying a very potent instrument in preventing and combating body odor; this eventually enables you to have a complete sense of comfort and also make you confident in social circumstances.

Whenever you have confidence that you are totally free from the menace of body odor, it becomes very easy for you to start a conversation with new people with a complete sense of optimism and maintain positive social relationships.

Personal hygiene is a lifestyle that places your physical, mental and social wellness above every other thing, not just only about the way you look. There is a great significance to the seemingly insignificant act of personal cleanliness that we perform every day.

It is quite evident that you can actually live a prolonged, fuller and a more fulfilled life by learning what it requires, and making a good use of it to your benefit. Therefore, practice good hygiene, since it is an art form that has the capacity to change your life for better.

Adopting these useful and essential habits will definitely result in several advantages, not just for you alone but also for those around you.

Chapter Four

UNDERSTANDING YOUR GENETIC NATURE

What is Genetic Nature?

Genetic nature in this context has to do with family health information, conditions and diseases about you and your close family relatives.

A proper understanding of your family's health history may have a very strong influence on knowing your risks of developing hereditary conditions and diseases.

Maybe you have possibly at one time or the other heard someone commenting on a similar health characteristic that you share with a family member, or perhaps heard people saying someone is the carbon copy of another family member.

It is an absolute truth that family members share homogeneous appearance; however, beyond that, family members also share gene, which are not really easily seen.

Just take for example; you may never be aware that you also share one of your great grandparent's increased risks for particular diseases.

Thus when it concerns the issue of wellness, having a proper knowledge of your family's traits that you can't see is optimally essential because, it may be an indication to the fact that you are at the risk of certain condition or illness.

This is one of the reasons why it is very needful to build a robust family health history. This can easily give quick solutions to your health risks and make provision for your care team to have a more complete picture of your health issues.

Some of the high risk of hereditary health conditions and disease, that is, the health conditions that flow include the followings:

    a. Heart Disease
    b. Stroke
    c. Diabetes
    d. Certain Cancers
    e. Depression
    f. Arthritis
    g. Asthma
    h. Dementia
    i. Osteoporosis
    j. Hernia

Majority of these above listed health conditions can be almost entirely dependent on genetic inheritance from your progenitors.

For instance, if you have a close family member who has breast cancer, your tendency for developing that same type of cancer is very high; especially when one or more of your close family member has had the disease in the past.

However, having a proper understanding of your family health history can go a long way in promptly alerting you and your health care providers, to the areas where you might be at a greater risk than the general population.

Forming A Family Health Record

Properly documenting your family health records doesn't need to be stressful in any way. Let it commence by discussing with close family members about their health and make sure it is properly documented by writing it down or it can also be electronically documented in one place.

But you have to make sure the information is properly updated from time to time. For instance, find out if:

They have experienced any critical health challenges in the past or of recent.

If that is the case, then find out further when exactly and how did they occur?

Find out exactly how old was the great grandparents when they died, and what was the cause of the death?

One of the most suitable opportunities for asking such questions is at a family get together; or by creating a special time to ask your parents some of these key questions that will give you some clues on how to address certain health conditions that may be peculiar to your family bloodline.

This might help you to learn and discover something new, and everyone will eventually benefit from your discovery by better understanding and managing their vulnerability to certain health risks.

It will be of great advantage when you include information from about three generations of biological relatives, including children, siblings, parents, aunts and uncles, grandparents and cousins.

In the process of trying to gather these vital information, endeavor to be sure that your family health history include:

i.   Certain critical medical cases that can be inherited

ii.   Endeavor to ascertain the particular age at which they were diagnosed.

iii.   Also try to find out the common age at which people die and the likely common cause of death

iv.   Find out about how people are affected by the environmental factors, habits and behaviors such as use of tobacco, alcohol, working in factory with certain exposure to health risks etc.

Ethnic Background

You may be little bit surprised at this juncture and begin to wonder what has environment and racial backgrounds to do in this regards.

Research has shown that families with the same culture and tradition are most likely to reflect a common characteristic. Moreover, various studies have revealed that some illnesses and conditions are more common in certain ethnic and racial groups than others.

For instance, African- Americans are at a greater risk of contracting sickle cell anemia; Caucasians are at the higher risk of cystic fibrosis. Asians have a higher risk for tuberculosis, and Hispanics have a higher risk of cardiovascular disease.

The Essence Of The Information

It is evident that information is a highly essential key in life; therefore when you have acquired the right information about your family health history, what then is the next thing to do with the information? This is very important.

Note that it is of a very great significance for you to ensure that the information of your family health history is properly stored in a safe place.

Moreover, it is also very essential that you make copies of the information to be shared with some of your family members, so as to make it convenient for them to also assess their risks. You must as well make it available for your healthcare givers.

Together, you can discuss what risks have been discovered and what should be the necessary steps to be taken to decrease them.

It is more likely that your health care provider may decide to prescribe some of the following steps for lowering your vulnerabilities:

i.   *Change Of Lifestyle*

Your care providers may consider certain adjustments in some of your built up habits and behaviors in response to your higher risks as great significance by delaying or, in some instances completely prevent disease.

ii.   *Conducting Screenings*

Conducting certain medical examinations, such as mammograms, blood sugar tests or colonoscopy, may be recommended at an earlier age or more frequently if your family history points to a higher risk of certain conditions.

A frequent genetic counseling in some instances could also be of great help and may be recommended.

iii.   Preemptive Treatments

Where and when it is the need arise and it becomes absolutely necessary, preemptive treatments such as the intake of calcium and vitamin D supplements if you're at a higher risk for osteoporosis may be recommended.

It is worthy of note that your family knowing family history alone, is not enough to determine if you will develop a disease or not. However, having the information readily with you puts you ahead of the game and helps you to be prepared to take proactive steps as regards your health.

You and the team of your health care providers can effectively utilize your health information as an instrument to evaluate your risks and then do something proactive about it.

Chapter Five

ENVIRONMENTAL HEALTH

A general healthy environment is a very vital factor needed in achieving and equally sustaining healthy living. A safety and healthy environment is one of the foundations upon which a healthy and a qualitative life can be achieved.

To be able to achieve and equally enjoy a healthy living, a healthy environment must be guaranteed. The quality of the environment in which you find yourself will determine the quality of your health life.

You can't enjoy a safe and healthy life beyond the level to which your environment is safe and healthy. In essence, to a large extent, a healthy environment is equal to a healthy life.

A quality and safe water, having access to a well balance diet, living in a pollution and noise free environment, etc. All these contribute immensely to man's general wellbeing and healthy living.

The quality of where people reside and the nature of their connection to their immediate environment can drastically affect their physical and mental health.

Environmental health is the public health department that supervises and regulates physical, chemical, and biological factors that impact human health. Although, it is quite evident that most of these environmental factors are sometimes out of control.

Precisely, environmental health is the area of public health that has to do with all the various ways the environment can affect physical and mental wellness of humanity.

Some of the things that have the capability of impacting your health adversely in your environment include the following:

1. Air Quality

It is quite clear that air is highly essential to human existence. Evidently, quality air is absolutely non-negotiable for human existence. Quality air is fundamental for human survival, and it can have highly essential effects general wellness of man.

 Negative air quality had been connected to a very great proportion of health challenges, such as the lung cancer and chronic obstructive pulmonary disease.

Research has also revealed that poor air quality is to a large extent caused by people's act of indiscriminate act of burning and waste disposal.

For example, in a particular research that was conducted, it was discovered that air pollution was connected to low birth weight in infants.

That is according to the research, it was discovered that the people were opened to an excessive amount of air pollution at the early and towards the late stages of their pregnancy were at a very high risk of having babies with lower birth weights, compared with those that were not exposed to air pollution.

2. Water Sanitation

According to a report by the Center for Disease Control and prevention, an estimated seven hundred and eighty (780) million people worldwide, don't have access to safe drinking water.

Therefore, it's important to note that, the simple act of boiling, filtering and chlorinating your water before consumption will definitely go a very long way in preventing water related diseases like typhoid.

3. Toxic Substances And Hazardous Water

According to toxicology, that is the field of science that is committed to knowing how chemicals and substances can impact people and their environments.

Majority of the substances needed for the advancement of industries and technology, like heavy metals or even plastics, can also affect the human systems and subsequently result to complicating health challenges.

It is therefore of great importance for you to consistently imbibe the consciousness of the adverse effects of the impacts of these substances to your general health.

4. Industrial Estates

For the primary purpose of safeguarding your overall wellbeing, and also for the purpose of the avoidance of contamination of dangerous diseases that are associated with toxic substances like industrial smokes, metals and plastics, it is advisable to always ensure that you avoid staying in a very close proximity to the locations of such industries with hazardous tendencies.

5. Waste Management

Improper waste management policy is another area of health challenge that authorities of various societies must not take with levity in order to ensure that people's health is properly safeguarded.

Indiscriminate waste disposal and management constitutes a great health hazards to the society. It is one of the major ways by which the air we breathe in is contaminated. This also has a way of polluting water, food and the general environmental safety.

Therefore, a proper approach to proper waste management must be adopted in order to achieve reduction of the high risk of contracting infectious diseases that are associated with improper waste disposal and management.

6. Noise

It is an undeniable fact that noisy environments also have a way of affecting human physical and psychological health in a negative way.

Therefore, when operating heavy noisy machines, it is advisable that you use gadgets that will reduce the impacts of the noise on your ear.

It is highly important that those who unavoidably live and work in noisy atmospheres need to always take precautionary steps to ensure safeguarding their health.

Chapter Six

REGULAR EXERCISE

What is Exercise?

Exercise can be defined as any conscious movement of your body that makes your muscles function and enable your body to burn calories. Exercise is any form of physical activities that keeps you active, energetic and healthy.

Regular exercise has been shown to help boost energy levels and enhance your mood. It has also been proved that regular exercise is also connected with other numerous health advantages such as helping in reducing susceptibility to contracting serious illnesses.

There are various kinds of exercises involving physical activities such as swimming, running, jugging, walking, among many others.

Making yourself engaged with the mind set of exercise has been proved to have numerous health advantages, including physical and mentally. Regular exercise has a way of making you look healthy and also guarantees longevity.

The following are some of the different ways in which regular exercise can be of immense advantage to your body and brain:

1. Weight Management

Being passive for a long time can have a great role to play on weight gain and obesity, and this can subsequently result to debilitating health challenges.

Regularly engaging yourself in exercises will culminate in enabling you to control your body weight which is very essential to your overall health.

Those who constantly indulge in the habit of regular exercises have a very low risk of developing obesity compared with those who don't indulge in the practice of regular exercise.

Your body consumes energy through exercise in the following ways, they are:

i. Proper Food Digestion

Food digestion in human body requires energy which in most cases is derived from both your conscious and unconscious exercises. That is to say, the required energy that the human body needs in achieving proper food digestion is referred to as exercise.

Although, the energy required for proper food digestion may not actually be limited to the conventional exercises of running, swimming, or jugging, nevertheless, it is obvious that a certain level of exercises take place in achieving proper food digestion in human body.

ii.*Heartbeat And Breathing*

Your normal heartbeat is highly essential to your general wellness. Your proper breathing and normal heartbeat determines how well blood is pumped from your heart through your arteries, and flow to the different parts of your body.

This process also requires energy, which is derived from regular exercises, and this eventually results in achieving the proper functioning of all the body parts.

2. Exercise Creates a Sense Of Enthusiasm

According to studies, it has been revealed that regular exercise is one of the ways by which you can improve your mood and reduce a sense of despondency, worries and despair.

In a particular research conducted on how exercise affects one's mood, it was discovered that about ten to thirty minutes of exercise is enough to meaningfully improve your mood.

Exercise has the capability of increasing your brain functionality from serotonin and nor-epinephrine.

These hormones have the ability to relieve feelings of depression.

Regular exercise also has the ability extend the creation of endorphins, which enables to create positive moods and decrease the feelings of pain. Your negligence to exercise may affect your mood in a negative way.

In a review conducted some time ago, it was found that people who suddenly stop the habit or regular exercise constantly come across major developments in symptoms of stress and perplexity, just within a couple of weeks.

3. Exercise Increases Vitality

Regular exercise has a way of enabling you to improve your strength while at the same time enabling you to decrease general body weakness. This may also double as therapeutic plan if you have certain health challenges like cancer and waste pain.

Aerobic exercise has the capability of ameliorating your cardiovascular system and also improving lungs health in particular.

The more you are active, the more your heart pumps more blood, this eventually translate into enabling your heart to release enough oxygen to your functional muscles.

Through your consistent exercise, your heart is enabled to be productive in transporting moderate oxygen into your blood.

Regular exercise leads to minimal pressure on your lungs.

4. Reduction Of Your Risk Of Chronic Diseases

Research has proven that constantly indulging in physical activity is a highly essential key in minimizing your vulnerability to some health problems:

a. Type 2 diabetes
b. Cardiovascular diseases
c. Different Cancer cases such as: colorectal, breast, and liver cancer among other types.
d. High cholesterol
e. Hypertension.

5. Exercise Is Good For Muscles And Bones

The fact that exercise plays a vital role in building and sustaining strong muscles and bones cannot be over emphasized.

The more people grow older, the more they are exposed to the possibility of losing muscle mass, energy, and activeness. This eventually results to making people to be at higher possibilities for injury.

Therefore, maintaining the habit of regular exercise becomes necessary for reduction of muscle loss and keeping yourself strong as you grow older.

Regular activeness also enables you in building bone density, which is a key contributive factor to a healthy and energetic living.

Some group of Researchers some time ago discovered that constant activeness has a way of improving bone density in the lumbar spine, neck and hip bones in a significant way. This has the possibility of enabling you to avoid osteoporosis later in life.

The positive effects of regular exercises like gymnastics, running, jugging or soccer have a great tendency of promoting stronger bone density compared with other sports like swimming and cycling.

6. Exercise Can Improve Sexuality

Take note that sexuality in this context is exclusively restricted to the married couples. Indulgence in any form of sexual relationship with someone you are not legally married to is an act of immorality.

That been said, research has proved that regular exercise has a way of impacting your sex life in a positive way.

Many marital crises are as a result of unhealthy and boring sex life. However, this menace can be properly addressed with the help of regular exercises, especially on the part of the husbands.

For instance, research has shown that engaging in regular exercise can improve your heart's strength; it can also enhance blood circulation into the various part of the body.

Regular exercise can enable you to achieve flexibility in your body, and all these will eventually result in enabling you to improve your sexuality, and subsequently help in curbing sex related crises in the home.

In several researches that have been conducted, there have been consistent results that exercising regularly for a long period of time has the capability of enhancing erectile functionality in men.

In addition to that, another study also revealed that the habit of constant exercise can result in enhancing sexual excitement, pleasure and general wellness in women.

7. Exercise Enhances Pain Alleviation

In many cases, certain chronic pains can be highly demoralizing. For decades, the prescription that was constantly recommended for the treatment of severe pains was rest.

According to some studies conducted by a group of researchers some years back, they came out with the recommendations that engaging in aerobic exercise can provide natural reliefs for pains and consequently enhance quality of life.

One of the ways by which engaging in regular exercise may help to avert or minimize severe pain is as a result of the fact that enables you to bear pain over time.

Regular activity can enable you to manage pain related with the different health challenges such as:

    a. Debilitating low back pain

b. Fibromyalgia

c. Serious soft tissue shoulder disorder

8. Exercise Is Essential To Skin Health

Your skin can be impacted by the quantity of oxidative pressure in your body. Oxidative pressure usually takes place when your body's anti-oxidant immune system is no more able to comprehensively renew the cell impairment occasioned by composite regarded as free radicals.

This in some instances result to the destruction of the cells formation and lead to having adverse effects on your skin.

This oxidative stress that is not really needed in the body system can be eliminated through constant engagement in intense physical activities.

In a study conducted some time ago, it was reliably revealed that constant physical activities regular exercise can result in slowing down the manifestation of skin aging and also avert psoriasis.

9. Exercise Helps Brain Health And Memory

Another important function of regular exercise is that it has the capability of enabling your brain perform optimally and at the same time safe guard your recapitulating and reasoning abilities.

It is evident that physical activities have the ability of enhancing your heartbeat rate, and this eventually results in enabling the smooth flow of blood and oxygen to your brain.

Regular exercise also serves as stimulants for the secretion of the hormones that are in charge of promoting the growth of brain cells.

Take for instance, regular physical activities have been proven to be responsible for the growth in size of hippocampus, and this has been of great advantage for improvement of mental functions. This is an aspect of the brain that is responsible for recapitulation and studying.

Consistent conscious exercise is highly significant in older people in the sense that it has a way of enabling to reduce the psychological effects of your brain.

Regular physical exercise is undoubtedly of great significance because it can also be of great help in reducing changes in the brain that can add to certain health challenges such as Alzheimer's disease and dementia.

10.   Relaxation And Sleep Quality

Another vital aspect of life in which exercise is necessary is because it has the tendencies of enabling you to achieve good relaxation and have a good sleep.

Regular exercise can enable you to enhance your sleeping quality because the energy loss that takes place while exercise invigorates constructive procedures during sleep.

A particular research conducted for a period of over four months in people with serious sleeplessness discovered that, both stretching and resistance exercise are useful in enhancing sleep quality and length of time; and at the same time reduces length of time it takes to fall sleep.

Exercise offers incredible benefits that can improve nearly every aspect of your health. Regular physical activity can significantly increase the production of hormones that make you feel happier and make you sleep better

Chapter Seven

ESSENTIALS OF MEDICAL CHECKUPS

Oftentimes, most especially when you are still much younger, you feel medical checkups are of less significance and you therefore easily decide to put off appointments with your primary health care provider.

Nevertheless, the mere fact that you're feeling well does not imply you should all together neglect the habit of periodic medical checkups with your primary health care givers.

The act of going through a periodic medical checkup that's most applicable to your overall wellness is highly essential for your overall healthy living.

What Are Medical Checkups

Checkups are the appointments you have with your health care providers, not because you are necessarily sick, but to ascertain whether there is a prospect of any kind of illness in your body system.

Where and when there is proper awareness, you don't really need to wait until you fall sick before you start running helter-skelter after your care givers.

The fear of being diagnosed of having a particular illness or lack of funds should not be excuse for regular medical checkups.

Regular checkups helps you to keep recommended screenings up to date and also helps in identifying problems as early as possible.

The more you regularly communicate with your primary health care providers, and allow them to be fully acquainted with how you are feeling and taking care of your body, the better chance they have of identifying and helping you avoid health challenges.

The time frame between checkups may vary depending on age difference, risk factor for health problems, etc. In some cases, your health care provider may be in the better position to determine the frequency of checkups that is most suitable for individuals.

For instance, high blood pressure is often referred to as "silent killer" because in most cases, there are no symptoms. The first symptom of high blood pressure can be a disastrous case like a heart attack, stroke or even sudden death.

Blood pressure checkups are routine checkups, providing your primary health care provider with a history of your normal blood pressure ranges. Routine checkups also help identify and strop problems before they develop.

If you suffer from a chronic illness, you might need additional checkups. You can't manage a chronic health condition well without appropriate checkups with your health care team.

This may not always be your physician, sometimes it may be another member of the team.

Essentials of Medical Checkups

Medical checkups are highly essential in three major ways:

It helps to determine if there is a prospect or a possibility of any health issue, and then find a way of preventing it before it develops.

Secondly, in the case whereby there is there is a particular health issues in your family history, which you as a member of that family may be vulnerable to, you then begin to take necessary steps that are required to ensuring preventing it, or you start to learn how to manage such issues if they can't be prevented.

Thirdly, routine checkups help you immensely in developing the skills that are required for the management of certain health conditions after they have been discovered at early stage, through the process of routine checkups.

A routine appointment for checkups is a perfect time to exhaustively interact with your primary care provider, giving them the necessary insights into your needs, both for the present and also for the future.

The duration of the time you spend with primary health care provider is exclusively determined by the nature of your needs.

Be Plain With Your Care Givers

Taking the full advantage of the opportunity, it is highly essential to patiently have a great session of dialogue about your health, ensuring you divulge every mystery that may be of help to your primary health care provider in finding a lasting solution to your health issues.

It is totally unwise and absolutely unnecessary to keep any sensitive information about your own personal health challenge, or any information about your family health history, while discussing with your health issues with your health care providers.

In some instances, in order to enable your care providers properly ascertain the problem, they may recommend different forms of medical examinations such as blood screening, x-ray, scanning, or other laboratory tests.

Regular medical checkups play a vital role in attaining and also maintaining your overall wellbeing, and in identifying potential health challenges at an early stage before they develop, degenerate and eventually get out of control.

Medical checkups are of great importance in the sense that they are very powerful tools for the long term preservation of both physical and psychological health, as well as serving as a key component in the prevention and treatment strategy of various ailments.

The Importance of Regular Checkups
i. *Early Detection Of Health Challenges*

One of the major roles that regular medical checkups play is that of assisting medical practitioners to discover potential diseases as early as possible.

This includes early discovery of chronic health challenges like hypertension, diabetes, heart diseases, and certain types of cancer.

It is evident that early discovery of those killer diseases through medical checkups profoundly enhances the possibilities timely treatment with optimal results.

It is therefore highly advisable that you should not for any reason whatsoever underrate the relevance of periodic medical checkups.

This will definitely go a very long way in guaranteeing your overall health, and also help to prevent potential health related challenges from degenerating and getting out of hand.

ii. Provision For Preventive Measures

It is obvious that medical checkups are not just merely instruments for early disease discovery. Rather regular checkups also serve as strong tools for curbing different health challenges from occurring.

Medical checkups are highly essential in the sense that apart from early detection of disease, prevention from certain disease can also be made possible. That is, medical checkup is basically a tool for disease prevention.

While achieving prevention of disease through regular checkups, the following factors are considered:

iii. Risk Factor Assessment:

Your health care providers will bank on your medical checkups to determine where you as a person could be at risk of certain health challenges. This may include trying to ascertain your genetic nature, exposure to alcohol and smoking habits, determining your diet, and other negative habits.

iv. Life Style Recommendation:

After a critical cross examination of the outcome of your medical checkups, your health care provider may decide to prescribe a particular adjustment in your lifestyle.

These lifestyle adjustment recommendations may involve the need for you to ensure dependence on balance diets; it may also include the need to engage in regular exercises, and also advices on how to manage certain health challenges.

The major reason for this kind of recommendations is primarily aimed at making sure there is a meaningful decline in the possibility of having certain particular health challenges.

v. Personalized Approach:

Periodic medical checkups enable health care givers to create personalized   health maintenance and statics for averting health challenges for every patient.

Take for instance, in a case where someone has been discovered to be a potential diabetic patient after checkups; your health care givers can recommend a certain degree for regular observation blood sugar levels and a change in your diet.

v. Changes Observations

Periodic medical examinations also help to make the determination in the variations in the nature of your health from time to time and also in observing the effects of the measures already applied.

In a situation whereby a change of certain lifestyle results in deterioration or improvement, then it becomes necessary for the care giver to adjust prescription and treatment methods.

Essentially, the fact that preventive medical examination is a very vital instrument for maintaining your general wellness and also a very reliable tool that one can always depend on for minimizing the tendency of contracting different kinds of illness cannot be over emphasized.

vii.   **Evaluation Of Existing Conditions**

With regards to those who already have been confirmed for having certain medical challenges, the diagnosis is never a death sentence; rather there is great hope for such people as periodic medical checkups play a very vital role.

In this case of medical examinations, it requires an intense observation and assessing the patient's present health conditions.

Up to date medical examinations enable health care providers to determine the effects of the applied treatment on the patient and help in discovering the areas where adjustments in the treatment strategy may be required.

Through the outcome of medical examinations, health care givers are able to access risk tendencies and possible complications with regards to certain medical situations.

In this case, it becomes very helpful for you to take the necessary proactive steps for prevention and also for quick intervention when the need arises.

Following the information that had been reliably gathered obtained from the checkups, health care providers are able to make available personalized prescriptions therapy, case management, and most importantly, proper compliance with the treatment prescription.

This is greatly helpful in the way illnesses are controlled and also helps in improving the qualitative life of a patient.

Furthermore, periodic medical tests have the capability of tacking overall health issues of complications; and it is quite obvious that when a health issue is detected at an early stage, coupled with how it is addressed with professionalism, it results in drastic decrease of the tendency of contracting chronic health challenges.

Essentially, proper observation existing health challenges by the way observing periodic medical checkups helps in achieving a productive and individualized care, this is highly essential in the management of the health of people with highly debilitating health conditions.

viii. *Life* Style Consultation

Within the scope of periodic medical examinations, medical professionals are able to offer resourceful counsels with the view of enhancing your habits and eventually your general wellness.

This particular mode of consultation through medical checkups offers a significant function in achieving your consistent healthy living.

It enables health care givers to evaluate your eating habits and they may decide to suggest prescriptions for enhancing the quality of your diets.

Such suggestions could comprise direction on the essentials of balancing macronutrients and micronutrients; it may also include the need for adjustment in the quantity of food consumption, completely doing away with diets that are not health for your system, and the need for focusing only on the foods that are enriched with the necessary nutrients.

Based on the result of your health records and your present medical status, your physicians may suggest particular measure of exercise such as mild sporting activities, taking a walk, and any kind of exercise that can enhance wellness that is suitable for you.

One of the major purposes of this recommendation is to enable you in taking a wise resolution as regards some of your habits that may have tendency of exposing you to certain degrees of health problems.

An adequate awareness of how a balanced died, indulgence in consistent exercises, and the knowledge of how to control certain health issues have the capacity to boost your wellness, makes these consultations a very significant part of medical examinations.

ix. Aging Management

The more we grow older, the more we begin to encounter certain transformations in our body, in order to properly control these body transformations that come with aging, regular medical checkups have important parts to play.

As far as this is concerned, medical checkup does not merely help in early discovery of illnesses, it rather play a very vital role in helping to control the health challenges that are related with advancement in age.

Aging is associated with an enhanced tendency of contracting different types of acute illnesses and health condition that has to do with key body organs like the liver, heart, lungs and kidney.

Medical checkups facilitates proper examination of these key body organs, it helps in recognizing the changes that have occurred as a result of aging, and makes it possible to provide suitable steps to enhance their function.

As you advance in age, regular medical checkups become more important to your health, and also for ensuring prevention from contracting certain preventable diseases.

The following points are the reasons why medical checkups become highly essential for age management:

i. Risk Observation

As you advance in age, you are faced with an increased possibility of developing tendency for incurring certain health challenges like diabetes, obesity, high blood pressure and also high cholesterol levels.

Placing yourself on a regular medical checkup will go a long way in enabling you to manage the tendencies and apply the required procedures to decrease the vulnerability of chronic diseases.

Regular medical examinations help in controlling these factors and in taking steps to reduce the risks of severe illness.

ii. Treatment And Prevention Plan

Regular medical checkups help in creating personal modes of therapy and tactics for preventing certain health conditions for a group of older people within a certain age range.

This may have to do with recommending a specific treatment plan, adjustment in particular habits, the need for exercise, balanced diet, diagnosis to detect illness at an early state and vaccination where the need arises.

iii. Functionality Management

As people begin to advance in age, you will observe that their ability to move freely, their flexibility of muscle, proper balancing, eyesight, hearing ability and other areas of the body that require optimal functioning may begin to decrease.

With the help of regular medical checkups, one is able to discover areas where decline has set in and begin to properly take the necessary steps needed for physical restoration processes to ensure normal functioning of the affected parts of the body.

iv. Mental Wellness

As aging begin to set in, one might begin to experience certain mental challenges that are associated with aging such as depression and worries.

In this case medical checkups could focus mainly on examining the psychological health and help to discover the main problem and recommend the proper treatment plans.

Essentially, regular medical checkups in adults focus majorly at attaining qualitative life, ensuring immunity from possible areas of complications and making it possible for people to remain active, attain healthy old age and without necessarily having to depend on others for anything but doing most things by oneself.

Chapter Eight

THE EFFECTS OF BAD HABITS ON HEALTH

Habits are the things you are engaged with in life that become part of your daily life. Some of these habits are highly essential to your overall healthy living.

While some of them could impact negatively on your health, especially when they are negative, and in some cases can even lead to serious complication, incapacitation or even sudden death.

I.   Alcohol

It is quite evident that indulgence in excessive consumption of alcohol, which could be either a single time consumption or consumption as a result of built up habit, can result to incurring chronic health conditions in your life.

Many people have lost their lives prematurely due to indulgence in excessive consumption of alcohol.

This is a very negative habit which its effects is not just limited health problems, but could also occasion wrong decisions, and in some cases excessive intake of alcohol can lead to deadly accidents in case of driving or operating machines.

The following are some of the areas of life whereby your health can be adversely impacted as a result of excessive intake of alcohol:

a. *Effects On Immune System*

Excessive consumption of alcohol can reduce the functionality of your immune system; this can eventually result to making your body to become weak in resistance to attacks and targets of illness.

The people that are addicted to alcohol are at higher risk of being infected with health challenges like pneumonia and tuberculosis compared with those who are not used to excessive intake of alcohol.

When someone drink too much of alcohol at a single time, it ultimately results in completely reducing his system's capability of fighting against infectious diseases.

b. *Effects On Brian*

Alcohol consumption disrupts the brain function channels; it can also alter the shape and functions of the brain.

The interruption of the brain system caused by excessive intake of alcohol can eventually result in alteration of mood and character, making it very difficult to reason in a proper way and also affecting one's ability to properly control oneself.

This might result to staggering and even falling, because one can no more control himself.

c. *Effects Of Alcohol On Your Heart*

Excess consumption of alcohol whether for a long period of time or drinking excessively for a short period of time can impact your heart's health negatively and this may result to incurring serious heart problems like:

1. Cardiomyopathy: That is the hearty condition where the heart muscles enlarge and the heart begin to malfunction.

2. Arrhythmias: This is a heart condition where the heart is no more breathing normally.

3. Stroke: This is the paralysis of some part of the body; and this could be partial or severe case of paralysis.

4. High Blood Pressure: This is another serious health condition of the heart that often results to sudden death or stroke.

d. *Effects Of Alcohol On Liver*

It is quite obvious from studies that drinking excessively can have negative effects on your liver. This can consequently result to different health conditions and liver enlargement such as:

* Fatty liver

*. Alcoholic hepatitis

*. Fibrosis

*. Cirrhosis

e. *Effects Of Alcohol On Pancreas:*

Excessive alcohol in the body systems result to making the pancreas to manufacture toxic matter which can consequently result to a health condition called pancreatitis.

This is a very chronic enlargement in the pancreas that results to a very serious inflammation and pain.

This condition affects the capability of the pancreas to produce enzymes and hormones that are highly essential for making food to adequately digest.

f. *Alcohol Causes Cancer*

Based on research, it has been unanimously proven that excessive consumption of alcohol can result in various kinds of cancer cases.

In an emerged result from a particular research, it was discovered that there is a correlation between alcohol consumption and increased tendency of contracting specific kinds of cancer.

In an emerged report from a particular research, it was discovered that there is a correlation between alcohol consumption and increased risk of certain types of cancer such like:

i.   Head and neck cancer, including oral cavity, pharynx, and larynx cancers.

ii.   Esophageal cancer, particularly esophageal squamous cell carcinoma.

iii.   In addition, people who inherit a deficiency in an enzyme that metabolizes alcohol have been found to have substantially squamous cell carcinoma if they consume alcohol.

iv.   Liver cancer.

v.   Breast cancer. A little drink of alcohol according to research can result to increase in women's risk for breast cancer compared to women who don't drink alcohol at all.

II.   Smoking Habit

This is the unhealthy habit of ingurgitating smoke from burning substance. The act of smoking occurs when you take in smoke from a particular burning substance through the mouth into your airways such as the lungs and eventually exhale it through your mouth and nostrils.

In many cases, those substances are dried leaves from tobacco, which have been processed in to cigarettes. While in some other instances, many people smoke the unprocessed locally planted tobacco leaves.

More so, in some other cases, people smoke a very dangerous herb which has many names to different people ranging from marijuana, weed, ganger, Indian hemp, etc.

The smoke from any of these substances go into your mouth and move down your air ways into your lungs and then begin to circulate in your blood vessels, it then begin to flow into your brain and eventually flood other body organs.

This substance is also referred to as Nicotine; this is a poisonous substance in tobacco that makes it difficult for people to stop smoking cigarettes.

The people who indulge in the habit of taking cigarettes hide under different guises for taking it, including claiming that smoking cigarettes helps their brain to create a calmness and enjoyment, and this is one of the reasons why it becomes very difficult for them to stop smoking.

However, it is quite evident that consuming cigarettes makes you to become highly vulnerable to some critical health conditions like cancer, stroke, cardiovascular disease, lungs disease and other health challenges that can be prevented by desisting from smoking.

III.   The Habit of Drug Misuse

This is another negative habit in which people get themselves entangled and find it difficult to be liberated, even when it becomes glaring to them that they have been badly hurt by the negative lifestyle.

Drug misuse can take place in different ways, for instance:

Drug misuse occurs when you decide not to follow up with your doctor's prescription for a particular treatment procedure for a particular health condition.

Drug misuse has taken place when your physician prescribes that you should take two tablets three times a day for one week, but you decide on your own to take one tablet once in a day for just three days against the physician's prescription.

This kind of action will result to making such health condition to develop resistance to treatment and eventually the health condition will become more complicated.

On the other hand, when your doctor prescribes that you should take one tablet once in a day and you decide on your own to increase the dosage against your physician's prescription, and begin to take two tablets three times a day, because you want to get a quick result, this could be very harmful to your health at the end, this is also a drug misuse, it is a habit that is very dangerous to your overall wellness.

Drug misuse takes place when you take hard drugs such as heroin, stimulants, cocaine, methamphetamines, marijuana, etc.

The habit of indiscriminately embarking on self-medication and taking drugs without a doctor's prescription is also an act of drug misuse; this can eventually be greatly inimical to your overall wellness.

Many people spend their lifetimes in rehabilitation centers, while many others end up in jail, all because of drug misuse.

Drug misuse has negative impacts on the entire human health but it basically starts its negative functions on the mental health, which could result to various mental health conditions such as:

a. Worries:

A heightened measure of brain chemicals through drug misuse has the tendency to cause increase in people's worries levels.

b. Brain Disorder:

Misuse of drugs and its consequences on the brain have the capacity of damaging one's reasoning capability and psychological objectivity.

c. **Memory Distortion**:

Continuous misuse of drug may result to impairment in one's ability to remember things properly. These may affect the ability to recall things that took place in the past and even the ability to retain things that took place in the recent time.

d. **Mood Swings:**

The variation in the degrees of brain chemicals occasioned by misuse of drugs can result in needless and meaningless swings in people's approaches to things.

e. **Changes Of Human Nature:**

When people take hard drugs or normal drugs in high dosages, it result in making them high, this consequently results in making them to feel and act differently compared with when they did not take those drugs.

This is one of the reasons people do unexpected and unimaginable things under the influence of drug misuse.

When this misuse of drugs becomes an addiction, it results in total alteration of people's real personality.

Misuse of drugs as an addiction leads to the alteration of the brain chemical levels, worries, frustration and other psychological changes that determines the way you behave and relate with people and react to situations on the daily basis.

Additional Effects Of Drug Misuse

Constant indulgence in the negative habit of misuse of drugs has a lot consequences connected to it.

The various consequences of drug misuse can be different based on different individuals, their general wellness, the kind of drugs they misuse, the frequency of the misuse of the drugs, and also the duration of the misuse.

Drug misuse cases should not for any reason be taken with levity because the consequences have ability of affecting general wellness, and in some instances it could even result in untimely death.

Potential effects of The people who indulge in the unhealthy habit of drug misuse are at higher risks of various forms of health challenges like: Weakened Immune System, Nausea, Vomiting, Involuntary weight loss, Arrhythmias', Blood vessel infections, Collapse veins, Cardiovascular diseases, Seizures, Stroke, Liver damage, Lung damage, Increased risk of infection, Hormonal imbalances, Conception issues, Miscarriage or Still birth.

IV.   Over Feeding

This is a habit that is underrated but must be controlled in order to avoid its overall negative effects on your general wellness. Eating a large or excessive quantity of meal can affect your health in numerous ways.

In some cases, over feeding is as a result of how the mail is so delicious, but in some cases it could be as a result of negative attitudes towards food, while some other instances, it could be an act of indiscipline.

Naturally, when your stomach is gauged it is very easy to know without anyone telling you that you are full, especially as an adult.

Over feeding when you continue to eat beyond the point of fullness. This can eventually result to adding weight against your wishes and adding extra weight makes you to become exposed to the tendency of developing health challenges.

Overfeeding has the tendency of making your belly to enlarge above it real volume to in order to make it adjust to the additional quantity of food.

When your belly begin to expand in order to enable it adjust to contain excess foods, it results in affecting other organs in your body; and consequently you become restless.

The restlessness caused by the enlargement of your stomach to adjust to food intake can eventually result to weakness, apathy and overall tiredness of the body. Take note of the following:

i.   When you eat excessively, it results in forcing your digestive organs to over function. Overfeeding results in making your digestive organs to produce more hormones and enzymes for the food to be appropriately broken down for adequate digestion.

ii.   In order to enable food to be properly broken down and made ready for digestion, the stomach generates a body chemical called hydrochloric acid.

iii. When you take excessive food, this hydrochloric acid may become congested in the esophagus and thereby causing heartburn.

iv.   The habit of taking excessive food that is rich in fats, such as pizza and cheese burgers has a high propensity of experiencing a health condition known as heartburn.

v.   When you eat excessively, it could also result in making your stomach to become gaseous; and this may eventually lead to a state of total discomfort.

vi.   Consuming excessive food is unhealthy because it can result in increasing your metabolism in the process of trying to consume the intake of excess calories.

vii.   This could consummate in in making you to experiment a partial sense of hotness, which may consequently lead to perspiration and a whirling sensation in the head with a tendency of falling.

Naturally when you eat, when you consume normal and moderate quantity of meal, your body system utilizes part of the calories in the food you consume for energy, while the other parts are deposited as fat.

When you therefore consume excess quantity of calories compared with what your burns, this may result to making you to experience unnecessary and unhealthy fatness, which have the tendency of cancer and other debilitating health challenges.

V.   The Habit of Sexual Immorality

Originally, sexual intercourse was exclusively designed by God for legally married couples. It is an undeniable fact that in this our contemporary world, sexual relationship has been grossly abused.

Sometimes one begin to wonder when you hear people make nasty comments such as saying they have lost count of the number of people they have slept with.

In most cases, people who indulge themselves in such indiscriminate sexual habits feel it's a way of proving their sexuality, and see nothing wrong with it.

However, it's quite evident that the unhealthy habit of immoral sexual act with a person to whom you are not legally married can have numerous negative implications.

The immoral habit of indiscriminate sexual intercourse with numerous partners has both short term and long term negative consequences. These consequences are ranging from both the physical health challenges, and also psychological problems.

Realizing that certain chronic sexually transmitted health problems like HIV and others have communicated from mothers to their innocent infants during pregnancy or during child birth is highly demoralizing.

This and many other sexually transmitted infections can be prevented to barest minimum if people can avoid the negative habit of indiscriminate sex and strictly stick to safe sex habit.

Majorly among the signs of sexually transmitted diseases are some of the followings:

1. Experiencing painful sore or bumps in the male or female private parts like the vagina, penis or anus.
2. Having difficulty and chronic pains in passing urine.
3. Irregular and abnormal emission of fluids from the penis or vagina.

    4. Abnormal emission of smelling fluids from the vagina.
    5. Abnormal bleeding from the female genitals.
    6. Irregular menstruation.
    7. Abnormal pains during sexual intercourse.
    8. Feverish conditions.
    9. Inexplicable rashes all over the body.
    10. Lower abdominal pain, etc.

In some instances depending on the nature of the health issue of individuals, some of the symptoms of the infections that are contacted through indiscriminate sexual intercourse may manifest just within a couple of days after contracting it.

However, in some other cases, there may be no significant immediate symptom, yet the infection could be silently creating damages in the body systems.

For instance, in many cases of gonorrhea, especially in the males, it does not take so long to be noticed when it is contracted, while in females, they may not feel any symptom or pain at all because they are only carriers.

Complications:

The complications these of sexually transmitted infections vary depending on individuals, but the most common ones include the followings:

a. Chronic pains in the pelvic region.
b. Various forms of complication in conception.
c. Swollen and painful eyes.

d. Chronic joint pains.

e. Swellings in the pelvic regions.

f. Different degrees of infertility.

g. Cardiovascular diseases

h. Different types of cancer cases like pelvic related, cervical and rectal cancers.

Steps For Preventions

There are many health challenges that can be prevented to a very large extent, including different types of sexually transmitted diseases. To avoid the risks of contracting sexually transmitted diseases, you have to:

i. Avoid indiscriminate sexual intercourse as much as possible.

ii. Stay with your spouse and your spouse alone, this may sound very stupid to some people, but this will be very helpful for you. Stop the negative habit of going about to have sex with everyone available and think you're enjoying yourself.

iii. It is reasonable to go for screening before marriage, most especially for those who might have been exposed to sex before getting married.

iv.   Ensure male circumcision, it has a way or reducing the risk of sexually transmitted infections.

Those men that don't circumcise are at greater risks of contracting sexually transmitted infections during sex compared with those who are circumcised, therefore circumcision is essential in helping to keep you from contacting sexually transmitted diseases.

VI.   The Habit Of Sleep Deprivation

There are certain things like not having enough sleep that you underestimate when it comes to the issue of health, but can have enormous negative effects on your overall wellness.

Sleep is part of God's design for the process of making the body to be fully repaired and reorganized after it has been broken and weakened through the normal daily activities.

Sleep is the process by which your body is made to reserve and gather strength. Thus you have to understand that when your body is prevented from having adequate sleeping time, the body has as well been prevented from the process of been able to accumulate and reserve energy.

This consequently causes the body to begin to experience weakness and makes it ineffective in its functions.

However, when the body is given adequate and sufficient time to sleep, it enables it to amend and adjust from the strength and vigor it has lost in the course of daily functions.

Essentially, when the body is deprived of having sufficient sleep, it eventually causes the body to become unable to perform self-maintenance and restoration that is required for adequate and maximal operation.

More so, adequate sleep is what enables the body to have sufficient rest that makes it possible for the relaxation and optimal functioning of the brain.

Adequate sleep is highly essential for the proper and optimal functioning of every organs of the body, and the brain is not exempted.

When you have adequate sleep, it enables your body to help in adequately re-organizing nutrients in the body system. It also helps to naturally detoxify your body systems and revitalize it for optimal functioning in the activities of the following day.

Studies have revealed that disrupting your sleep routine with up to one or two hours may have negative effects on your feelings, thereby causing temporal health challenges like:

Improper coordination, memory impairment, mood swings, anxieties, lethargy and withdrawal from routine functions.

Impacts of Sleep Deprivation:

When you don't sleep enough, it results to general weakness of the body and lack of strength.

a. Sudden swings in mood and psychological health challenges.
b. Lack of proper balancing and ability to coordinate well.
c. Memory Challenges and mental issues.
d. Sleep deprivation can result in vision impairment.
e. It can increase your level of worries and affect the way you respond to situations.
f. Lack of adequate sleep can reflect in change in your facial looks. It can reflect in making you look pale, it can affect the color of your eyes by making it reddish; it can also result in weight reduction.
g. Sleep deprivation may result to weakening your overall immunity against illnesses.
h. Sleep deprivation has a risk for increasing depression.
i. It can result to accident while operating a machine or when you drive.
j. Sleep deprivation has the capability to prompt high blood pressure and other cardiovascular diseases.

Chapter Nine

SAFE DIETARY HABITS

The quality of what goes into your body system such as food or drinks, is highly essential to your all round wellness. Therefore, there is a need to always ensure the safety of your health by consistently being conscious of what you eat or drink.

Your body needs a variety of food to give you energy and keep your body functioning effectively.

That means eating a balanced diet that contains vitamins, mineral, and fiber, which can be found in fruits and vegetables, especially the leafy greens, whole grains, legumes, nuts, lean protein, and low fat dairy.

The healthy dietary that translate into living a healthy life requires your full concentration on consuming real foods.

To properly achieve living a healthy life, you must cultivate the habit of living on unprocessed foods.

It is always safe and healthy for you to eat a combination of both animals and vegetable plants like: Meat, fish, eggs, vegetables, fruits, nuts, seeds as well as healthy fat oils and high-fat dairy products.

For those who are physically sound and also strong, with natural and normal weight size, without any form of health challenge, if you eat unprocessed carbohydrates moderately, there is no challenge.

Such carbohydrates include potatoes, sweet potatoes, legumes and whole grains such as oats.

Nevertheless, for those who are having extra weight, and have manifested certain symptoms of metabolic cases such as diabetes, it is wise for them to completely desist from some major souses of carbohydrates, and they will see their health improving naturally.

Studies have that the act of simply reducing intake of carbohydrates by eating less can help people to reduce their weight. It is highly essential that you watch what you consume, especially when it has become obvious that such foods can trigger health challenges in your life.

Some Foods That You Must Avoid

Some of these foods that you need to avoid in order to safe guard your health are substances that have been associated with various adverse health conditions, and should therefore be completely avoided or minimized.

In some cases, you discover that people are even addicted to some of these food items, even when they are fully aware of the negative effects that such foods constitute to their general wellness.

1. *Monosodium Glutamate*

This is a very popular substance that is used as supplements in food for the purpose of increasing the natural flavor of the food. A majority of refined foods such as frozen dinners, salty snacks and canned soups contain a certain measure of this food additive.

Many restaurants and fast food centers make use of a certain quantity of monosodium glutamate in the course of processing their foods.

There is an emerged argument about its negative effects on human brain when it is consumed in a large quantity.

2. *Artificial Food Coloring*

Artificial food coloring is used to brighten and improve the appearance of everything from candies to condiments.

In recent times, there have been many concerns as regard their potential health effects. Concerns also have been raised about the potential cancer causing effects of certain food dyes.

A report showed that artificial coloring may promote hyperactivity in children, although another study showed that some children may be more sensitive than others.

Food dyes are primarily found in processed foods, which should be limited in healthy diet. Always opt for whole foods, which are higher in important nutrients and naturally free of artificial food coloring.

3. *Sodium Nitrite*

Sodium nitrite is frequently found in processed meats. Sodium nitrite acts as preservative to prevent the growth of bacteria, while also adding a salty flavor and reddish pink color.

When exposed to high heat in the presence of amino acids, nitrites can turn into nitrosamine, a chemical compound that can have negative effects on human health.

4. *Guar Gum*

Guar gum is a substance obtained from endosperm of guar seeds and used especially as thickening agents to thicken and bind foods.

It is widely used in food industries and can be found in ice cream, salad dressing, sauces and syrups. It is high in fiber and has been associated with a multitude of health benefits.

A study shows that guar gum can be helpful in reducing the symptoms of irritable bowel syndrome such as bloating and constipation.

Another research also reveals that it may also help to lower blood pressure and cholesterol levels. However, high quantity of guar gum may have adverse effects on human health.

5. *High Fructose Corn Syrup*

This is a sweetener made from corn. It is often found in soda, juice, candy, breakfast cereals and snack foods. It is rich in a type of simple sugar called fructose, which can cause serious health issues when consumed in high amounts.

Particularly, high fructose corn syrup has been linked to weight gain, and diabetes. Additionally, high fructose corn syrup contributes empty calories and minerals that your body needs.

It is therefore best to skip sugary snacks and foods that contain high fructose corn syrup, which may have negative effects on your general wellness.

Go for whole, unprocessed foods without added sugar, and sweeten them up with fresh fruits.

6. *Artificial Sweeteners*

Artificial sweeteners are used in many diet foods and beverages to enhance sweetness while reducing calorie content. Some common types of artificial sweeteners include aspartame, sucralose and saccharine.

Generally, artificial sweeteners are considered as safe for most people when consumed in moderation.

However, if you experience any negative effects after using artificial sweeteners, check ingredients labels carefully and limit your intake or completely avoid it as the case may be.

The fact that a particular substance is safe for one person's consumption does not necessarily imply it is equally safe for your consumption.

7. *Sodium Benzoate*

Sodium benzoate is a preservative often added to carbonated drinks and acidic foods like salad dressings, pickles, fruit juices and condiments.

As good and essential it may be, studies have uncovered some potential side effects that should be considered when combined with vitamin C.

Sodium benzoate can also be converted into benzene, a chemical compound that may be associated with cancer development.

Carbonated beverages contain the highest concentration of benzene, and diet or sugar free beverages are more prone to benzene formation.

It is highly essential for you to always avoid foods that contain ingredients like benzoic acid, benzene or benzoate, especially if combined with a source of vitamin C, such as citric acid or ascorbic acid.

8. *Artificial Flavoring*

Artificial flavors are chemicals designed to imitate the taste of other ingredients. They can be used to imitate a variety of different flavors, from popcorn and caramel to fruit and beyond.

Studies have shown that these artificial flavors can have some worrying side effects on health.

A study that was conducted on animals concerning artificial flavor showed that grape, plum and orange synthetic flavorings inhibited cell division and were toxic to bone marrow cells.

Therefore, always look for "chocolate" or "cocoa" on the ingredients labels rather than "chocolate flavoring" or "artificial flavoring".

9. *Yeast Extract*

Yeast extract, also called autolysed yeast extract or hydrolyzed yeast extract, is added to certain savory foods like cheese, soy sauce and salty snacks to boost the flavor.

It is made by a combination of sugar and yeast in a warm environment, then spinning it in a centrifuge and discarding the cell walls of the yeast.

It contains glutamate, which is a type of natural occurring amino acid found in many foods. Much like monosodium glutamate, eating foods with glutamate may cause mild symptoms like headache, numbness and swelling in people who are sensitive to its effects.

Yeast extract is relatively high in sodium, with about 400 milligrams in each teaspoon. Reducing sodium intake has been shown to help decrease blood pressure, especially in people who have high blood pressure.

10. *Food Poison*

Sometimes, farmers and food vendors are erroneously more conscious about the necessity for the preservation of their harvested food crops and preventing them from being destroyed by post-harvest pests like weevils and the likes.

However, it is absolutely wrong for anyone to be conscious of preserving food crops more than the way they are conscious of the hazards of some of the chemicals they use for preservation on the immediate and remote effects on human health.

As much as it is highly essential for farmers to preserve their crops from being destroyed by post-harvest pests, we must always take to cognizance the importance of the safety of the health and the lives of the people that will eventually consume such products.

The farmers and food vendors who need to preserve their food products should also remember that the safety of the health and lives of the final consumers of the crops should also be properly taking into consideration.

Many people have lost their lives while many people's health have been adversely affected as a result of indiscriminate use of unfriendly and unhealthy chemicals for preserving food items by farmers and also by food vendors.

11. *Wrong Eating Times*

Many people don't understand the reality of the fact that eating wrongly, such as not eating on time is as bad as eating unhealthy food. Studies have revealed that the unhealthy habit of frequently skipping of breakfast is responsible for a vast proportion of stomach ulcer cases.

Those who habitually skip breakfast are prone to developing stomach ulcer, especially when they engage themselves in laborious activities. These are health challenges that can be completely avoided but have led to untimely deaths.

In the same vein, the unhealthy habit of eating very late in the night and going to bed immediately is also responsible for many health challenges that people grapple with from time to time.

Research also reveal that the habit of eating very late in the night without getting involved in any physical activities is responsible for many cases of indigestion, heart burn, constipation, stomach pain, insomnia etc.

Ideal Eating Periods

*Breakfast*____7:00 am-8:00 am. It's not wrong to eat between thirty minutes to one hour after waking up. However, it is absolutely unhealthy to be habitually having your breakfast later than 10:00 am

Lunch____12 noon to 2:00 pm. It is ideal to eat within four hours intervals between breakfast, lunch and dinner. Taking your lunch later than 4:00 pm is considered as having skipped your lunch and that should be taken as dinner.

Dinner_______________________________________6:00 pm to 9:00 pm. It is proper to have your dinner between these periods. Eating two to three hours before going to bed is ideal. It will help in facilitating proper digestion and prevent cases of indigestion, hearth burn and constipation.

Conclusion

Going by the example of how man lived a healthy life, completely void of any form of health challenge while he was in still the Garden of Eden, it is quite evident that God is still interested in the attainment of the overall wellbeing of mankind.

However, due to certain seemingly prevailing factors, man has always found it difficult to achieve and sustain a life of total healthy living.

Never the less, most of the factors that are responsible for man's inability to achieve a life of complete healthy living, coupled with continuous battles against all manner of health challenges, are absolutely under the control of man.

Man is therefore left with the option of either applying the keys that guarantee attaining and also sustaining a healthy living and seeing the expected results, or neglecting the proper application of the keys and continue to grapple with various health challenges that could have been prevented or well managed.

This highly resourceful book has revealed that healthy living is absolutely achievable when you do the things that are expected to be done.

When you adopt a lifestyle of safety consciousness, and begin to do all the other things that are expected to be done on your own part, it's evident that results would definitely be inevitable.

Safety consciousness is essentially the bedrock of achieving and equally sustaining a healthy living. Therefore, safety consciousness should not be considered as an event, it should rather be seen as an integral part of your daily life.

9 798300 481094